TREATING JOINT PAIN

A PATIENT'S GUIDE TO PLATELET-RICH PLASMA

AMIT MIRCHANDANI M.D.

Texas Cell Institute
8380 Warren Pkwy #201, Frisco, TX 75034

For bulk ordering and rights permissions requests, please visit http://www.texascellinstitute.com.

First Edition.
ISBN 978-1542743006

26 25 24 23 22 21 20 19 18 17   1 2 3 4 5 6 7 8 9

MEDICAL DISCLAIMER

While every effort has been made to ensure the information in this book is complete and accurate at the time of writing, no warranty is made that it is free from errors, or up-to-date.

Nothing in this book is intended as individual medical advice, nor should it be taken as such. No book is a substitute for a detailed consultation and/or examination by a physician. You should not attempt to diagnose or treat any disorder based solely on the contents of this, or any other, book.

Any products mentioned in this book are recommended only after seeking advice from a qualified physician. All matters regarding your health require careful, personalized and individualized medical attention.

Neither the author nor the publisher may be held liable for any damage, loss, or injury sustained by anyone who relies solely on the information provided in this book or on information from websites, articles, books, organizations, or any other medical practitioners who may be mentioned in this book.

No person associated with this book is responsible if a reader decides to seek help from an insufficiently trained physician in the field of regenerative medicine.

"The doctor of the future will give no medicine but will interest his patients in the care of the human frame, in diet and in the cause and prevention of disease."

-   Thomas Edison

Table of Contents

FOREWORD

As an early adopter of biologic alternatives, in my medical practice I have seen the explosive growth in the use of Regenerative Medicine in the orthopedic marketplace.

I joined the Crane Clinic for Sports Medicine where platelet-rich plasma (PRP) was first adopted in 2005. Much maligned by fellow physicians for the use of this novel alternative to traditional surgical and pharmaceutical models, we were driven by our patients and their success stories. Providing new treatment options for patients suffering from chronic pain kept us striving to improve and advance the field of regenerative medicine. We could provide a pain-free life for so many patients, for whom more traditional medical interventions failed.

At Crane Clinic, we have trained over 75 physicians in the use of PRP.

PRP should be viewed as a viable option to the current chronic-pain management paradigm.

I met Dr. Amit Mirchandani through one of Bluetail's training opportunities. Since the visit, he has built a practice and frequently contacts us for collaboration and additional updates and specific learning cases. Dr. Mirchandani has shown a great passion and talent in this specialty of medicine. When Dr. Mirchandani shared with me his book, *Treating Joint Pain: A Patient's Guide to Platelet-Rich Plasma*, I was thrilled. As a respected physician in this growing specialty of medicine, he saw the need for a way to explain PRP to patients.

Treating Joint Pain: A Patient's Guide to Platelet-Rich Plasma outlines the traditional approach to pain management and how it often falls short in achieving a successful result. Dr. Mirchandani has included a detailed summary of those variables that affect healing such as diet, smoking, and stress. This book then moves on to discuss in detail PRP treatment.

Dr. Mirchandani gives an excellent summary of what exactly is a platelet, how these little cells work, and what exactly is PRP.

Patients and other interested individuals will find this book easy to read and informative. Although PRP is still considered "investigational" by most insurance companies, evidence to support its use in diseases such as tennis elbow, jumper's knee and early knee osteoarthritis have shown it to be safe and effective.

The Internet is a source of much disinformation about Regenerative Medicine. Add in to the mix all the "stem-cell" clinics popping up across the country with no protocols and outrageous claims. The situation leaves a patient at risk of becoming prey to unethical practitioners. I am glad to see a book that provides a practical source of information for patients as they consider this exciting new treatment option.

Kristin Suzanne Oliver, M.D., M.P.H

Co-Founder and Physician Partner

Bluetail Medical Group

St. Louis, Missouri 2016

"What we call biologics. They're on their way, and that will be a transformational event."

- Dr. James Andrews, world renowned Orthopedic Surgeon

"The ability to modulate the inflammatory cycle with interventions like platelet-rich plasma, may prove to be the most therapeutic breakthrough in arthritis management in recent times."

-Umar Burney, MD Founder, Orthopedic Specialists of Dallas World Renowned Joint Replacement Surgeon

PREFACE

I wrote *Treating Joint Pain* with my patients at the forefront of my mind. For years, patients have undergone millions of steroid injections, been prescribed a plethora of dangerous medications, and have had to rely on invasive surgery to help alleviate joint pain. Early in my career, I knew there was a hole in the options we were offering to patients. I had done thousands of steroid injections and written books of prescriptions, all before I even finished training.

The problem was that patients weren't always getting effective, definitive long-term pain relief. They would have periods of short-term relief, but then their symptoms would return, sometimes worse than before treatment started. Medications often gave partial relief, but often at a terrible cost of side effects and addiction to narcotics.

My instincts and the data right in front of my eyes told me that I must be able to provide better options for my patients. I had to think in terms of giving my patients regenerative, NOT degenerative options to help heal joint pain.

We are in trouble in America. Our patients are increasingly suffering from chronic pain, disability, and having to undergo surgery at alarming rates. We are spending over a trillion dollars a year on musculoskeletal disorders alone. We are right in the middle of a narcotic epidemic that is completely ruining and even taking the lives of our patients. This is the 30,000-foot view of what is going on in our country and I have founded my practice, Texas Cell Institute, to help patients with a regenerative, cellular-based approach to treating joint pain.

The regenerative approach is a process. It's not a magic pill or injection. It requires a commitment, a communication and mind-shift to a long-term solution instead of a quick-fix, short-lived treatment. Our patients at Texas Cell Institute have done well because we spend a lot of time and resources educating them about their injury and treatment options. We treat patients like our own family, following up as much as necessary to continuing improvement. We care about a patient's overall health- their diet, sleep, alcohol and tobacco use, their weight, exercise habits, sleep, and stress. We help them understand how these factors play a huge role in chronic pain and overall inflammation. We provide very focused physical therapy in conjunction with our potent and precise cellular-based interventions. It's an extremely effective process.

Platelet-rich plasma (PRP) is one of these cellular based interventions that has transformed the way we treat pain and injury. Its research is mounting and applications becoming more and more widespread. Our high-level athlete patients, who rely on their bodies have opted for PRP to get back to their sport with minimal downtime and joint preservation in mind. At Texas Cell Institute, we are committed to providing PRP at the very highest quality to give our patients the best chances for success.

I am very proud of what we have been able to accomplish at Texas Cell Institute for so many patients thus far, but our work is far from done. We must help millions of patients understand their options for joint pain and help them commit to a regenerative approach. We must help millions of patients to avoid committing to repetitive short term solutions, including long term steroid use and narcotic use. We must help millions of patients get better and live the life they were meant to live.

I thank you for picking up this book, for taking your valuable time to learn about treating joint pain and platelet-rich plasma. It is my hope and desire that I answer all your questions in this book, but if there are any more, don't hesitate to contact me directly.

ACKNOWLEDGEMENTS

Thank you, Roshni, for being my beautiful wife and everything you are to our family. You are my teammate, laughing partner, supporter, organizer, home manager, social planner and find time to be a stellar physician to those who suffer from HIV. Oh yeah, the best part — you're an absolutely amazing mom to our two loveable sons, Arav (3) and Krish (1).

Thank you to my incredible parents, Priya & Bobby Mirchandani, my very first teachers in life. You both have always taught me to help people in any way I possibly can. Even though it is not that big a deal, you both still have that glow in your eyes when you say your son is a doctor who helps people. Thank you for a life filled with unwavering support, guidance, advice, knowledge, and love.

INTRODUCTION

On January 18, 2009, Hines Ward of the Pittsburgh Steelers was leading his team to victory over the Baltimore Ravens in the AFC championship game when a tackle from Ravens cornerback Frank Walker twisted his leg in the grass. With the Super Bowl just two weeks away, the resulting medial collateral ligament (MCL) sprain to his knee could have been disastrous. Traditionally, an MCL sprain would put a player out of the game for a minimum of three weeks. Determined not to miss out, Ward opted for platelet-rich plasma (PRP) treatment to his MCL, which he credited with helping him to compete in the Super Bowl, where he was named the Most Valuable Player.

Since then, many other athletes have opted for PRP treatment to help heal injury. Other high-level professional athletes have used

PRP to heal their injuries, including Kobe Bryant, Tiger Woods, and L.A. Dodgers closer Takashi Saito. There are many examples of athletes using both PRP and other types of regenerative medicine, because they want to heal their bodies, not degenerate them with short-sighted pain management.

They want to avoid medications that could interfere with their concentration, and delay or eliminate the need for invasive surgery. PRP helped keep these professional athletes competing in their sport, with minimal time off from competition, and helps preserve their joints for long-term health.

I have treated some high-level and professional athletes, including B J Penn and Diego Sanchez, two UFC Fighters who flew into Dallas to get PRP treatment to help heal their painful joints before they started training for fights.

Stephen Curry is the 2015-16 Kia NBA Most Valuable Player. He had PRP therapy this year during the playoffs to help enable him to return to the court faster.

Although we can learn from athletes in how they approach injury, PRP is not only for athletes. It's for you, me, and potentially everyone who suffers from chronic nagging joint pain, non-healing injuries, and arthritis. Platelet-rich plasma is a cellular-based biological therapy gaining international recognition as a potentially game-changing treatment for healing joint pain.

For years, physicians have focused on merely managing joint pain, hoping to give patients enough relief to get by. If you are a patient who has suffered from chronic pain, your experience may have gone something like this: multiple doctor's visits, prescriptions, narcotics, steroid injections, ongoing therapy, and braces — collectively leaving you with partial, if any, long-term pain relief. This can be expensive, on your time off work, your wallet, your mood, and your overall quality of life. Then, when these treatments have failed to give long-term pain relief, you may have found that surgery was your only option. In the process, you may have also been told you must modify, and even give up, the activities or sports you once enjoyed.

Simple activities like walking, climbing the stairs, and working in the yard are no longer possible because of lingering pain. Dreams of playing sports with your kids and grandkids may disappear. Many patients are even forced to change their jobs to accommodate their chronic pain. The results of chronic pain may be a more sedentary lifestyle, weight gain, trouble sleeping, reliance on pain meds, disability and sadly, never getting back to the life you meant to live.

Joint pain should be taken seriously from the very first time you experience it. The body has an incredibly strong ability to heal most of our cuts, bruises, and painful injuries on its own in a matter of days to weeks. However, in certain circumstances, injuries don't heal and pain persists.

At this point, my recommendation to you is to commit to a regenerative approach to healing your injury, utilizing your body's own powerful cells and growth factors precisely directed to areas of injury. Platelet-rich plasma is an incredibly important regenerative treatment modality for you to consider if you have chronic, non-healing pain. Please read this book and you'll see why.

With a regenerative approach to chronic joint pain and injury, evidence is mounting that shows we can relieve pain, potentially regenerate damaged tissue, and definitively heal injury. By doing so, we decrease and eliminate the need for long term pill-popping, help you avoid surgery, and improve your overall wellness, energy, function, and activity. Our goal is not to merely manage your pain. It is to heal your injury and help you live the active, pain-free life you want to live.

So, what's the deal?

How come all physicians don't know about PRP and offer regenerative treatments to their patients?

Many of the answers to these questions lie in the depths of the infrastructure of modern medicine. The truth about modern medicine is that the business side of medicine has increasingly taken over the practical side. Let me explain so you are aware of the context.

Doctors and patients are not the only two pieces of the modern medicine puzzle. In fact, doctors and patients are becoming ever less influential in the scope of medical practice. The doctor-patient relationship, once at the core of medical practice, is now governed by which insurance company covers you, and which networks your doctor belongs to, or works for. Other players, like pharmaceutical companies, and device companies have increased their influence, determining pricing, and which therapies patients have access to.

Pharmaceutical companies can sometimes spend nearly a *billion* dollars for a drug to come to market. At that level of expenditure, they seek to regain their investment and may a) up the cost of their medication, and/or b) be incentivized to keep patients on their medications as long as possible, thus increasing the lifetime value of each patient.

In addition, doctors who practice preventative medicine, who choose to talk to patients at length about overall health and wellness, or who attempt to help their patients stay off medications, are often reimbursed significantly less for these efforts by insurance companies.

It is much easier and more profitable for physicians then to see more patients, spend less time with each, and prescribe medications instead of preventing disease by changing a patients' behavior, nutrition, and lifestyle. It's not the doctor's fault, however; it's the system at play.

If our system was interested in the health and wellness of our patients as a focal point, should we not properly reimburse prevention, nutrition, and non-invasive regenerative approaches for pain, to advocate driving down our country's overall medical costs? Is it strange that we continue to pay more and more into our healthcare system, but the people of our country keep getting sicker and more disabled?

Instead, some of our brightest doctors from the best institutions are going into procedure-driven sub-specialties rather than primary care and prevention, partially because the reimbursement is more favorable.

Again, it's not the doctor's fault; it's the system at play.

It is important to educate our patients to understand the current situation in modern medicine. Our main objective is to encourage you to take control of your own wellbeing, educate yourself on health and wellness, and seek options that preserve your health. We have written this book to help you understand one of those options in regards to chronic, non-healing joint pain — platelet-rich plasma — an effective, non-invasive way to help heal your chronic joint pain.

PRP and stem-cell therapy have changed the nature of what we can do, and the data and evidence is continuing to mount.

While there's a lot of press coverage and awareness raising for heart disease, cancer, and other major causes of death, it's much less reported that musculoskeletal disorders are the major cause of disability,[i] and account for more than half of the sick days lost to the US economy.[ii]

One in four Americans is diagnosed with a musculoskeletal condition yearly that requires medical treatment[iii]. There are numbers that suggest 18-20 million people in the United States have arthritis, and this number is on the rise due to our country's obesity epidemic and a baby boomer population that is living longer. We spend yearly $1trillion on joint problems in our country alone,[iv] and those numbers are rising. In fact, according to the Bone & Joint Initiative, spending on musculoskeletal disease equates to 5% of the GDP.[v]

It is important for the general health of the population to approach joint pain in a regenerative manner, preserve our innate joint symmetry, avoid surgery if possible, and increase our overall health and quality of life.

Don't get me wrong. I have a deep respect for what orthopedic surgery has done and continues to do for millions of patients. As a board-certified anesthesiologist, I witness successful surgeries on a weekly basis. Many patients would have lived much of their life with canes, crutches, and wheelchairs without surgical orthopedics. Yet, at the same time, I fully support and implement regenerative options prior to surgery, which can reverse painful symptoms, restore function, and potentially heal injured structures. As you will see, regenerative options have many important advantages over our current treatment options, including less recovery time and fewer side effects and complications.

So, we must take control of our health and go back to putting the patient-doctor relationship at the central core of how we practice medicine. We must first focus on wellness and prevention, on augmenting the body's own repair process, and on regenerative rather than degenerative treatments. We need to look longer and harder at the side-effects of accepted treatment paradigms, and extend the principles of "doing no harm" beyond the immediate, to include the long-term repercussions of certain treatments like prescription narcotics and soft tissue exposure to macro-dosages of steroids.

Platelet-rich plasma therapy can help regenerate your damaged tissue, and, combined with our comprehensive anti-inflammatory program, will potentially help you heal your joint pain and preserve your body from the harm of degenerative treatment modalities. Choosing the regenerative route to reversing joint pain may not only improve your pain and quality of life, it may also potentially save the entire medical industry, including you, tons of money.

UNDERSTANDING THE HEALING CASCADE

Blood is comprised of four components.

- ☑ Red Blood Cells (RBC's)
- ☑ White Blood Cells (WBC's)
- ☑ Platelets
- ☑ Plasma

These components all work together in various ways to accomplish multiple tasks. For instance, red blood cells deliver oxygen to all our tissues to keep those tissues and us, as humans, alive. White blood cells's are important in fighting infection and any foreign intruder into our body's system. **Platelets play a significant role in causing blood to clot (hemostasis) as well as releasing growth factors at areas of injury to initiate a healing process of damaged tissue.** Plasma is the liquid component of the blood in which all the other cells are suspended.

When an injury occurs, such as a cut on your skin, a ligament sprain, or even the wear and tear stress of cartilage in your joint, the healing response generally involves four overlapping phases.

☑ Hemostasis

☑ Inflammation

☑ Regeneration

☑ Remodeling

Immediately following a wound, platelets come to the scene of injury, clot blood if there is bleeding, and release very powerful bioactive growth factors at the area of injury, which leads to inflammation.

Inflammation can be good and bad. Acute inflammation, on one hand, is a critical part of the healing process. On the other hand, chronic inflammation can be a long-lasting, progressive, lingering pain that degrades a joint or soft tissue like cartilage over time.

The important thing to remember is that it is the activity of platelets which generally initiate and orchestrate the entire healing cascade. This is why platelet-*rich* plasma is so powerful.

The Phases of Healing

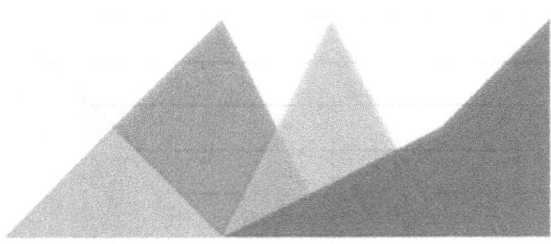

Time After Injury

Inflammation
(1 Hour -3 Days)
Wound Contraction
(3 Days- 1 Month)

Granulation
(8 Hours-10 Days)
Collagen accumulation
Remodeling
(3 Days - 3 Months)

Figure 1: The phases of healing in days after injury.

We will talk about what PRP exactly is, but in the meantime, understand that a high concentration of platelets at an area of injury can stimulate local inflammation, deposition of growth factors, the genesis of new blood vessels, and the recruitment of stem cells for the regeneration and strengthening of injured tissue.

So, platelets release the important growth factors for healing, which are powerful fertilizers at areas of injury. These growth factors then recruit stem cells (seeds) to areas of injury to differentiate into new, healthy tissue. Some of these growth factors released by platelets also help generate new blood vessels, to deliver nutrients and oxygen to the healing tissue as well.

THE PAIN MANAGEMENT PARADIGM

Much of the current joint pain treatment paradigm is based on faulty thinking. When we incur an injury, the affected area swells.

Swelling puts pressure on nerve endings, and results in painful sensations. These serve to warn us of the damage done, alert our body to protect the injury, and discourage further activity that could be harmful.

The problem is, inflammation hurts. So, even though we know it's a necessary part of the healing process, we try to prevent it, to reduce the pain.

Since healthy cells are not inflamed, the reasoning goes that by reducing inflammation, damaged cells will be restored to a healthy state. Or, at least, the pain will go away.

As we've just seen, though, inflammation is the vital first stage of the healing process. Interventions which disrupt the inflammatory process don't restore damaged cells to a healthy state. They simply delay or prevent the regeneration and remodeling necessary for healing to occur.

In the short term, anti-inflammatory medications do reduce pain. If you're focused on masking pain rather than healing, they work. This pain reduction comes at a cost, however - while masking pain in the short term, anti-inflammatories potentially reduce the body's ability to effectively heal the injured tissue.

The current approach towards joint pain, if rest, ice, compression and elevation fail, is to put patients on Non-Steroidal Anti-Inflammatory (NSAID) medication, which commonly have harmful side-effects, like stomach ulcers and even heart attack and stroke.

If NSAID's don't work, the patient often progresses to narcotics like hydrocodone. These can be very harmful to patients, especially when they are taken long-term. In fact, the Surgeon General has announced narcotic use is an epidemic in the United States. In parallel, patients often go on to injectables, such as steroids. Again, steroids also have side-effects, one of primary concern being cartilage degeneration. Not only do these medications not heal injury, but when taken long-term they may accelerate your need for more invasive treatment, such as surgery.

Let's take a brief look at these stages of treatment, at what's happening inside your body, so we can understand why focusing solely on short-term pain relief and reducing inflammation may not be the best approach.

RICE

Dr Gabe Mirkin introduced the Rest, Ice, Compression, Elevation protocol in *The Sports Medicine Book*[vi]. It quickly became standard practice, and was used by sports coaches and athletes for decades.

Typically, we can learn a lot from athletes and how they treat their bodies, because they rely on them to make their livelihood. They want to preserve their body; quickly and definitively find their diagnosis soon after injury; avoid long-term medication usage and, obviously, invasive surgery. They want to get back to their sport at a high level, and they want to do it without much, if any, activity modification or change in their level of intensity.

So, when the doctor who introduced the RICE protocol publicly revoked it in November 2010[vii] it caused some understandable confusion. As Dr Mirkin explains, "both Ice and complete Rest may delay healing, instead of helping."

The main problem is that healing requires inflammation, but cooling the area with ice delays it. What happens is that all the blood vessels in the area contract, and reduce blood flow to the injury, rather than just any ruptured vessels.

Even worse, unlike the cardiovascular system, which is powered by your heart pumping blood around your body, the lymphatic system has no pump. It's a one-way system that relies on capillary action to wick the lymph away. Cooling reduces the capillary action, and can result in the waste materials being sucked back into the interstitial spaces between cells in the injured area, instead of being carried away. That leaves you with a build-up of toxins, and slows the healing process.

Applying ice for prolonged periods can potentially do more harm than good, causing decreased effectiveness in your lymphatic system and a buildup of toxins at the area of injury, thus slowing the healing process. Prolonged ice to injury may also result in frost burn, and irreversibly damage surrounding tissues and nerves.

NSAIDs

It's not just ice that slows down the healing process, though. As Dr Mirkin says, "Anything that reduces inflammation also delays healing." That includes ice, NSAIDs, corticosteroids, and anything that blocks the immune system's natural inflammatory response.

Non-Steroidal Anti-Inflammatory drugs include Ibuprofen, Celebrex, Naproxin, and Aspirin. These are common first-line agents prescribed by primary care physicians and specialists. They're given to patients in the hope that some of the anti-inflammatory benefits will allow patients pain relief.

But NSAIDs don't only act on the injured area, and they're not only anti-inflammatory. Because they're ingested orally and introduced to the bloodstream, they affect your whole body in ways we still don't fully understand.

Most people think because they are easily available, and they are in prevalent use, that NSAIDs should be very safe. However, some of the more serious side-effects of these drugs are stomach ulcers, bleeding, kidney failure, and even liver failure. NSAIDs account for 3 to 9% of total drugs prescribed, but 25% of reported adverse drug reactions[viii].

Although NSAIDs can be used safely to a certain degree, just for the acute inflammatory phase, many times these medications are often used in a prolonged manner - sometimes every day for years, to treat a chronic condition. Obviously, the longer a patient takes NSAIDs, the higher the chances of side-effects developing become. Also, elderly patients, who typically have multiple prescriptions for potent drugs to deal with a range of health issues, are even more prone to adverse side-effects.

Side Effects of NSAIDs

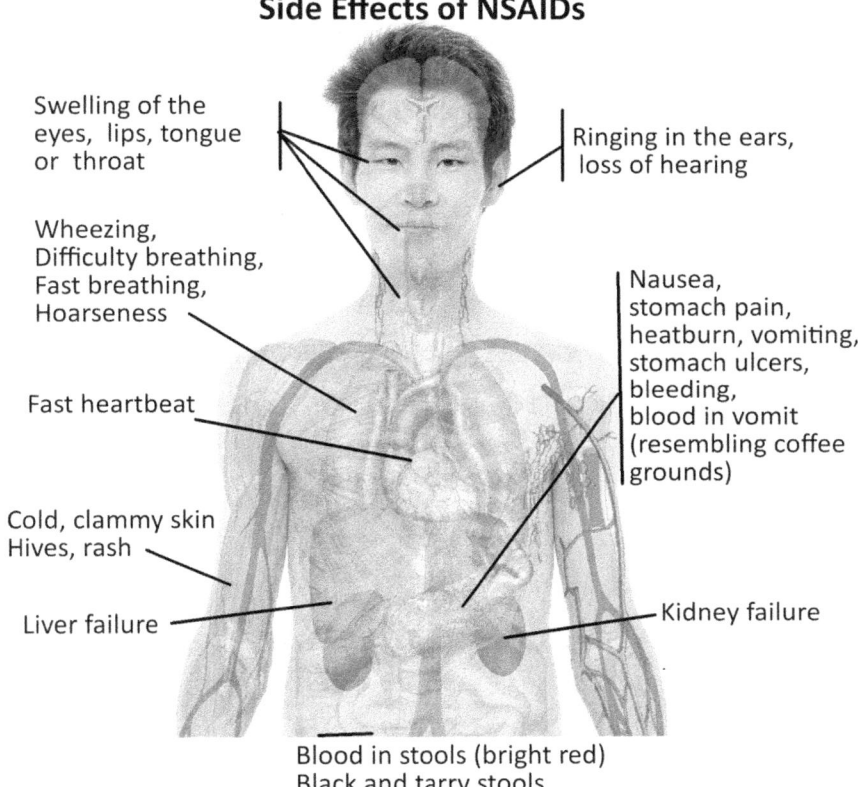

Swelling of the eyes, lips, tongue or throat

Ringing in the ears, loss of hearing

Wheezing, Difficulty breathing, Fast breathing, Hoarseness

Nausea, stomach pain, heatburn, vomiting, stomach ulcers, bleeding, blood in vomit (resembling coffee grounds)

Fast heartbeat

Cold, clammy skin Hives, rash

Liver failure

Kidney failure

Blood in stools (bright red) Black and tarry stools

Figure 2: The potential side-effects of NSAIDs

Even though NSAIDs can offer some pain relief, it comes at a high cost, especially if used in a prolonged manner.

In contrast, PRP can have a potent local anti-inflammatory effect without the potentially dangerous system-wide side effects.

Narcotics

When NSAIDs fail to provide sufficient pain relief, patients are prescribed opioid narcotics. Dr. Nora D. Volkow informed the Senate Caucus on International Narcotics Control in May 2014[ix], that:

> The number of prescriptions for opioids (like hydrocodone and oxycodone products) have escalated from around 76 million in 1991 to nearly 207 million in 2013, with the United States their biggest consumer globally, accounting for almost 100 percent of the world total for hydrocodone (e.g., Vicodin) and 81 percent for oxycodone (e.g., Percocet).

Some of the side-effects from these narcotics are common and include constipation, nausea, vomiting, drowsiness, and dry mouth. Narcotics can also can be very dangerous, and can cause respiratory depression, have powerful addictive properties, and can cause death.

Dr. Volkow reported an estimated "2.1 million people in the United States suffering from substance use disorders related to prescription opioid pain relievers in 2012."

There are several famous cases of people who have died from narcotic overuse. Most recently, Prince died after an accidental overdose of the opioid fentanyl. The problem isn't confined to the rich and famous, though.

Deaths related to drug poisoning due to opioid prescription in the US overtook those tied to heroin or cocaine abuse in 2002[x]. By 2014, prescription opioid deaths increased by 3.34 times to almost 20,000. That's over 75% of prescription drug-related deaths, and considerably more than heroin and cocaine combined[xi].

Just like NSAIDS, we prevalently prescribe opioids here in the United States for chronic pain. Sometimes the message is lost that just because these medicines are prescribed, it doesn't mean they are risk-free. Patients often don't understand the problems narcotics have the potential to cause.

During my early years in pain management, I saw firsthand the type of negative impact narcotics caused patients. It's a very difficult process to wean patients off narcotics once they are chronically on them. The beauty of

PRP and cellular-based therapies, is that patients can potentially avoid taking prescription medicine in the first place.

STEROIDS

Cortisone is a type of steroid. It is commonly injected as an anti-inflammatory agent, again to help reduce the patient's pain. Fortunately, steroids work quickly. Many times, patients walk out of a clinic appointment after a steroid injection feeling good already. However, the problem is that over time, repeated use of steroids can be associated with cartilage toxicity and soft tissue degeneration. The steroids themselves are toxic to cartilage cells, and are continuing to do damage to joints behind the scenes[xii].

A common storyline with patients who have received a series of steroid injections showcases a diminishing rate of return on each injection. Patients often return 3-4 weeks after a steroid injection saying, "that was great, but the pain has returned." Then with the second injection, they may say, "This one only lasted for a few weeks," and after the final injection of three, they may say, "That barely lasted at all, I was in pain the next day after I woke up."

As long ago as 2002, sports medicine experts who encouraged family physicians to undertake steroid injections as part of their practice warned, "There is some concern that corticosteroid preparations, with repeated use, may accelerate normal, aging-related articular cartilage atrophy or may weaken tendons or ligaments." [xiii]

In 2015, a systematic review of *The Effect of Intra-articular Corticosteroids on Articular Cartilage* by researchers at Stanford University concluded that "beneficial effects are supported for IA administration [of corticosteroids], but the lowest efficacious dose should be used," and that, "the long-term negative effects of these medications on articular cartilage has remained a concern." [xiv]

Steroid injections play a role in managing inflammation and joint related pain, however it is critically important to understand that steroids can also accelerate the degeneration we wish to halt. You will soon see why PRP may be a significantly better alternative to steroids in your path towards healing joint pain.

SURGERY

The final step in the pain management paradigm, when rest, ice, compression and elevation, bracing, NSAIDs, narcotics, and steroids have all failed, is commonly surgery.

Surgery has done many patients well in the history of modern medicine. Many surgeons are deservingly considered heroes in thousands of households across the world. Surgery, however, is commonly placed at a portion of the treatment spectrum, *after* all conservative options have been exhausted. The reasons for this are important to understand.

1. Surgery is an invasive procedure and introduces risk to the patient, including the risk of infection, bleeding, anesthesia, risk of allergy or rejection to implants, risk of damage to internal structures of your body, and – rarely - even death.
2. Surgery is expensive, both in terms of medical costs, and downtime for recovery.
3. With surgery, you may also burn bridges toward full healing and recovery. Surgeries that excise tissue, to help heal injury, undermine the bodies' natural scaffold. That

can mean causing asymmetries in your body and bypassing the bodies' capacity to heal itself. If you already have a joint replacement, for instance, you have already given up your capacity to apply regenerative medicine modalities and preserve your own joint.

4. The patient's range of movement may be restricted and activity modified. Their ability to carry out normal activities may be compromised; they may not be able to go back to playing tennis or golf, or go back to being a carpenter or a plumber. The patient's quality of life and even career potential might not be fully restored, even after surgery.

5. Finally, the number one side-effect of surgery is ... chronic pain. Imagine disrupting the bodies' innate symmetry and going back to square one. It is not uncommon for patients to continue to suffer from chronic pain and remain on narcotics after surgery.

Although surgery has its risks, despite our best efforts in helping heal injury, some patients will eventually need surgical intervention.

Surgery is a critically important option in our arsenal to treat musculoskeletal pain. It is important, however, to understand and exhaust regenerative treatment options prior to undergoing surgery.

THE HEALING

AUGMENTATION PARADIGM

Traditional approaches to pain management have hit a ceiling in terms of what they can offer patients with chronic joint pain. With these approaches, physicians often struggle to heal injury. Most treatment options can only mask painful symptoms, not identify and heal the source of injury.

The healing augmentation approach can work with the body's own powerful growth factors and regenerative cells, and reduce symptoms that have caused chronic nagging pain. But beyond that, regenerative therapies, such as platelet-rich plasma, can help facilitate long-term healing, and improve patients' quality of life.

PREVENTION

If you're already suffering with joint pain, you probably don't want to hear about how it may have been avoidable. At the same time, it's never too late to make lifestyle changes that could help slow your joints' degenerative process as well as decrease your body's over-all inflammation.

The field of Regenerative Medicine is not a series of magic therapies. It is simply a powerful approach based on decreasing inflammation, restoring the health of tissue at the cellular level, and healing injury. We harvest, isolate, and utilize powerful regenerative cells and growth factors to maximize your body's own ability to repair and heal itself. The precise delivery of these regenerative cells to areas of injury is critical, but still only a piece of the entire regenerative process. Lack of sleep, stress, diet, smoking, and other diseases such as diabetes can all significantly contribute to your joint pain as well.

Often, at Texas Cell Institute, we see patients whose localized joint pain may be due to chronic inflammation, for instance, but discover that much of their body is inflamed because of lifestyle decisions such as their diet and smoking. In response, we treat the whole body and give all our patients a program to help decrease their overall systemic inflammation, which also can help heal their specific joint pain as well. This program may include nutritional supplements, and even a formal nutritional consult. It might mean seeing other specialists, from sleep specialists for sleep apnea, smoking cessation classes, even fitness classes tailored specifically to their physical needs. We take great pride in the network of specialists we have built to help you in your regenerative path back to health.

Here, we'll look at the major contributing factors to body-wide inflammation, and some changes you can make to start to relieve your symptoms.

Diet & Nutrition

Did you know that what we eat and drink can cause joint inflammation? Our body's ability to heal begins with creating a healthy internal cellular environment. Your diet is a critical part in either causing inflammation and a degenerative cellular environment or helping you promote healing of inflammation, injury, and illness. The choices you make are incredibly important and we want to share some options with you to make your decisions simple and clear.

Food to Include

Fruit and Nuts:

Acai Berries

Almonds

Apples

Blackberries

Blueberries   Cashews

Flaxseeds

Lemon/Lime

Pine Nuts

Pineapple

Pecans

Pumpkin Seeds

Raspberries

Strawberries

Walnuts

Vegetables & Beans

Asparagus

Bell Peppers

Black Beans

Broccoli

Cabbage
Cauliflower
Celery
Cucumber
Eggplant
Garlic
Ginger Root
Green Beans
Kale

Kidney Beans
Leafy Greens
Lima Beans
Mushrooms
Radishes
Snap Peas
Sprouts
Zucchini

Fats & Dairy

Avocado Oil
Coconut Oil
Fish Oil

Flaxseed Oil
Goat's Cheese
Goat's Milk

Meats

Cage Free Eggs
Chicken
Fresh Fish

Lamb
Lean Beef
Turkey

Drinks

Black Coffee (limited)
Herbal Teas
Lemon Water

Mint Water
Purified Water
Raw   Vegetable
Juices

Herbal Supplements*

Aloe Vera	Omega 3
Bromelain	Peppermint Oil
Chondroitin	Traumeel (topical)
Fish Oil	Turmeric
Glucosamine	

*Always consult your physician or healthcare professional before using these supplements and let your doctor know the supplements you are taking.

Food to Exclude

As important as it is to eat good, healthy food, it is equally important to avoid food that's bad for you. The following foods are either poor in nutrition, may cause inflammation, or both. If you remember FAST MAGS, it will help you stay away from potentially harmful foods. Yes, it's tougher to do than to talk about, but you will reduce your body's overall inflammation and your body will thank you for it.

Fast Food–

Assume there is no healthy fast food choice

Aspartame-

An artificial sweetener, found in canned sodas

Sugar-

Anything that ends in −ose

Trans Fats

(Snack Foods, Frozen Foods, Donuts, Cookies)

MSG

Monosodium Glutamate, a flavoring found in most restaurant prepared food

Alcohol

Gluten,

A wheat protein (Pastas, Bagels, Crackers, Desserts, Breads)

Saturated Fats

(Pizza, Fast Food, Red Meat, Desserts)

Simple Steps to Take

- ☑ Use these food lists as a guide at the grocery store.
- ☑ Keep a food diary, so you can see what you're really eating.
- ☑ Avoid fast food and restaurants. Brown bag your lunch, and eat in as much as possible.
- ☑ Commit to the process.
- ☑ Reduce inflammation, heal your pain naturally, and reap the benefits.

We underestimate the importance of what we eat. We rarely relate what we eat to issues like joint pain. In the United States, we are heavy on fast food and prescription drugs. Neither of these are the answer to your joint pain. They are the problem.

Exercise & Activity

When we treat our professional athlete patients, our goal is to get them back to performing in their sport at a high level; to get them as healthy as possible as soon as possible. Although some injuries require a window of immobility and rest to help the healing process, as a rule exercise and movement has a strong anti-inflammatory effect on our entire body.

We also know that properly directed exercise helps to reduce and even reverse chronic systemic inflammation. That's why it's important to stay active and in motion; to chemically improve your body's ability to heal chronic inflammatory disorders, arthritic disease, and musculoskeletal injury.

The important thing is to commit to a body in motion. Something as simple as basic stretching daily can make an enormous difference in your body's response to injury. Ask those who do yoga on a regular basis how they feel - they feel well physically, mentally and emotionally. This is due to yoga's overall decrease in body inflammation.

Sleep

Pain and sleep are very closely connected. Poor sleep causes an increase in your body's total inflammation, which can then contribute to high blood pressure, weight gain, and other health issues, including joint pain. Poor sleep may also make your body more sensitive to pain and lower your pain threshold. This means poor sleep can increase your pain to otherwise non-painful stimuli.

Joint pain, ironically, may be the exact reason why you may have poor sleep to begin with. At least half of patients with osteoarthritis, for instance, have trouble either falling asleep or staying asleep throughout the night.

Sleep may also be disrupted by obstructive sleep apnea, stress, or even your specific sleep environment.

To improve sleep

☑ Do not eat a heavy meal before bed
☑ Avoid caffeinated beverages or alcohol before bed
☑ Avoid exercising late
☑ Avoid watching TV, or working in the bedroom
☑ Keep your bedroom comfortably cool, quiet, and dark
☑ Develop a bedtime routine and perform it every night
☑ Meditate prior to bedtime to decrease your level of stress

Smoking

Although everyone correlates smoking with lung disease and lung cancer, smoking decreases your body's healthy blood supply, and has a large role in musculoskeletal degeneration as well.

Smoking decreases blood supply to bones, ligaments, tendons, cartilage, and muscles. It slows the production of bone-forming cells, decreases the level of calcium absorption from your diet, and predisposes you to osteoporosis.

Smokers are much more likely to suffer overuse injuries such as tendonitis and bursitis. They have more severe musculoskeletal injuries when compared to nonsmokers, have a much more difficult time healing those injuries, have a higher complication rate after surgery, and a higher rate of infection and poor wound healing capabilities.

The good news is that many of these trends can be halted and significantly reversed with smoking cessation. If you want to commit to musculoskeletal health at the cellular level, it is important that you stop smoking.

But it can be a challenge to quit smoking, especially if you've had the habit for a long time. Here are some recommendations to help you.

- ☑ Join a Smoking Cessation Program to give you the support you need. Tell your friends and family you want to quit, and ask them to help you. Don't feel that you must, or even should, do it alone.
- ☑ Take vitamins, supplements and herbs – very often, medical detoxification works in synergy with smoking cessation.
- ☑ Hydration- water is a simple, available, cheap, and effective natural detoxifier that counteracts toxins such as nicotine.
- ☑ Increasing your level of activity and exercise
- ☑ Don't be too hard on yourself if you lapse. That will only make you feel bad about yourself, add to your stress, and make you more likely to lapse in the future. Instead, remind yourself that quitting is a process, not a one-time event.
- ☑ Replace smoking with a productive activity (i.e., 20 pushups)

Stress

Stress is mental and emotional, but it has physical implications as well, including inflammation. That same inflammation may cause your joints to swell, and lead to more pain with movement. Stress also can weaken your immune system, lead to muscle tension, muscle spasms, and stiffness that makes movement more difficult. This creates a downward spiral of more inflammation and pain.

To make things worse, stress reduces someone's tolerance for pain, so when you're stressed your threshold for pain may decrease significantly and you may have a heightened pain response. Finally, increased stress also can alter other choices we make, in terms of diet, alcohol, smoking and sleep habits, usually for the worse.

Breaking out of the stress cycle isn't easy. Much like stopping smoking, you might need help. There are things you can do yourself to start feeling better.

☑ Exercise causes your body to release endorphins, which decrease your perception of pain and reduce stress.

☑ Giving your mind an opportunity to release stress is an important strategy in reducing stress and promoting overall health. Meditation, yoga, and stretching can all help.

☑ Increasing your level of hydration improves cellular health, improves blood flow, decreases inflammation, and improves your immune system, improving your overall physical and mental health.

☑ Stress is a different challenge for everyone. Acknowledging your level of stress and seeking specifically tailored help is an important step in reducing it. Don't be afraid to consult your doctor or primary health care provider. Asking for help isn't a sign of weakness; it's a sign of strength.

SELF-CARE

For acute joint pain or injury, first stop the activity that caused it, and avoid putting any weight or strain on the affected joint. Have a medical practitioner examine you to see whether you have soft tissue, muscle, tendon, ligament, or bone injury. Your medical practitioner will direct your next steps of care. The initial aspects of care are focused on stabilization, protection of the injured area, and allowing the initial phase of healing to occur. Elevate the affected area to help with lymphatic drainage and reduce swelling.

Don't use any ice or heat treatments, and avoid analgesics if you can. Instead, immobilize injured bones, and apply light compression to injured soft tissues. Compression bandages can be used, but they shouldn't be tight enough to leave the surrounding area feeling numb.

Establish which movements cause pain or discomfort, and avoid them at first, but try to keep lymph flowing through the area by moving the surrounding areas. So, if your shoulder is damaged, you might be able to move your arm without pain. If your elbow is painful, you can wiggle your fingers to keep things flowing

Start with isometric exercises, where you tense the muscle without extending or contracting it.

REGENERATIVE MEDICINE

Regenerative medicine is an emerging field in both scientific research and in clinical medicine. This field which focuses on using your own body's powerful cells and growth factors to facilitate replacing or regenerating damaged or injured tissues to restore normal function after injury or disease.

Platelet-rich plasma and stem cell therapy, for example, remove, concentrate, and return your own cells precisely to areas of injury where repair must take place. One of the major advantages of these therapies is the opportunity to heal injury with virtually no chance of awful side effects, rejection, allergy, and life-time cost, which is often the case with prescription drugs. Instead, you are using your own body's platelets and growth factors to heal your injury, which essentially eliminates any possibility of rejection and even infection.

Regenerative medicine is, in one sense, a brand-new specialty. In another sense, it's the oldest we have ever had. It was our original specialty as human beings, before we had pharmaceuticals and fancy devices and a whole slew of medications being prescribed to us. We used to look for holistic ways to enhance healing, and use our own body's strong capacity to heal. So, in a way, medicine is coming full circle, but now with the immense technology and science behind optimizing our cellular capabilities to give your body the best chance of healing.

The specialty of regenerative medicine is growing, with pioneers in the field meeting together at national and international conferences and summits. We are in the process of creating educational platforms for patients and practitioners, and data registries to share powerful information and analytics amongst physicians who wish to help patients heal injury with regenerative medicine.

Pharmaceutical and device companies tend not to fund studies in regenerative medicine because, if the efficacy of cellular medicine is showcased, it could cannibalize their investments in selling drugs for disease.

Regenerative approaches to joint pain are also currently considered experimental by most insurance companies, but the research is developing and growing quickly. We are learning an incredible amount about how healing occurs on a cellular level, and how we can augment that. In time our regenerative approach to joint pain will become the norm, and be our first line approach. Some basic regenerative medicine therapies for degenerated joints include:

- ☑ **Platelet-rich plasma (PRP) and platelet-poor plasma** are created by drawing a small amount of blood, and separating the platelets from the other components using a centrifuge. The correct concentration of plasma and platelets for the specific injury are then verified and re-introduced at the site of damage via injection.
- ☑ **Bone marrow aspirate**, where stem cells are harvested from the bone marrow, processed and purified before being administered to damaged tissue. It is suitable for patients with advanced degenerative disease or injury that doesn't respond to platelet-rich plasma therapy.
- ☑ **Adipose-derived stem cell therapy** uses stem cells from your fatty tissues to promote the healing cascade.

PLATELET-RICH PLASMA

So, what is PRP and where does it fit into the Healing Augmentation Paradigm?

PRP is a cutting-edge, conservational, and minimally invasive approach to healing musculoskeletal injury. This is something that is truly preservative, something that directs treatment at the source of injury. It doesn't just mask the pain, but treats the source of injury, and can help regenerate that tissue.

It's a way of using the body's own properties, such that tissue can heal, with no long-term harmful side-effects, no long-term medication usage, no necessary interventions that will continue to degenerate tissue. It's a step towards decreasing medication use, increasing functionality and delaying or eliminating the need for surgery.

An Introduction to Platelets

We already talked about the role of platelets in our body. They're the short-lived, incomplete cell fragments without a nucleus that deliver the raw materials required for regeneration, which we call growth factors. Now, let's take a more in-depth look at what they are, what they do, and how they work.

We have known that platelets act in clotting for some time. We think of them as the cells that clot our blood after injury, so that we don't continue bleeding all over the place. However, we're constantly learning more about how the healing process works, and platelets are just as vital to the later stages of that process as they are in the early stages.

Platelets, like red blood cells, and most white blood cells, are created in the bone marrow. They come from large cells called megakaryocytes (that just means 'large nucleus cell') which break down into smaller chunks containing granules called alpha granules. It is in these alpha granules where packets of growth factors live.

These growth factors are very potent, and

powerful, in helping regenerate tissue. They're basically the building blocks other cells need, and they float around the blood stream in an inactive state until they receive a signal that tissue is injured, which activates them. Once activated, they travel to where they're needed, and get to work.

Platelets travel to the area of injury and initiate the entire regenerative process. First, they clot the blood, to stop bleeding. They also send out chemical signals that recruit stem cells and other necessary healing agents to the area. The growth factors they contain are responsible for cell division, new blood vessel and tissue formation, tissue repair, cell growth, collagen production, and hyaluronic acid production. They promote epithelial cell growth, activating and recruiting stem cells to areas of injury to regenerate new, healthy tissue.

As we learn more about platelets and their role in regeneration, it's possible that we may learn that regeneration is the primary function and clotting is a byproduct function. Really, it doesn't matter which is primary and secondary. The fact is that those functions work in concert and synergy with each other.

MAKING PLATELET-RICH PLASMA

Platelet-rich plasma is simply a volume of plasma (the liquid component of the blood in which all the other cells are suspended) that has a platelet count above that of your whole blood. Typically, what is defined as platelet-rich plasma is 5-7 times the base level content of platelets in your whole blood.

Normally, you have about 94% red blood cells, 6% platelets, and less than 1% white blood cells in your blood. When we create platelet-rich plasma, 94% of it is platelets; 6% is the other components, so we functionally flip the ratio.

We create platelet-rich plasma by drawing a small volume of blood, usually 60-90ml, just the same as we would draw blood for testing, or if you were donating blood. We take that blood to our certified lab, and with strict sterility, the blood is centrifuged, which means it's spun at a high speed to separate the blood components. The platelet-rich component is carefully isolated, properly assessed under a microscope and finally prepared for precise reinjection at the site of injury.

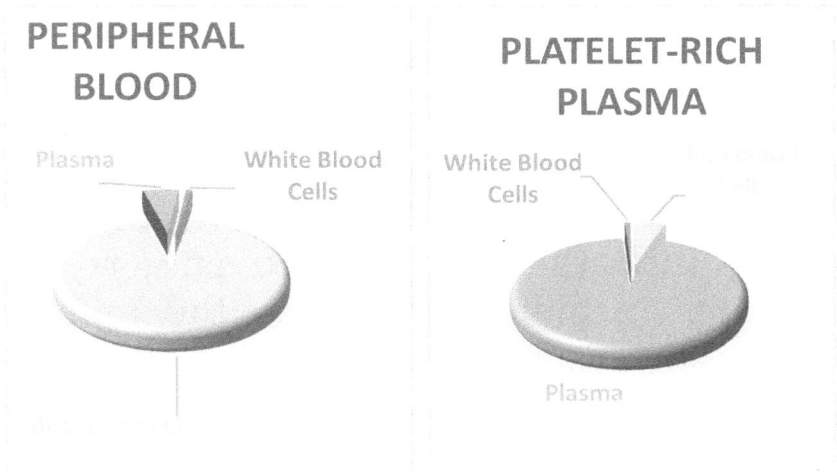

Figure 3: Cell ratios in normal blood versus platelet-rich plasma

There's no need to multiply or synthetically reproduce the platelets. PRP is a concentration of them. So, we're not introducing any foreign bodies that could upset the immune system, cause an allergic reaction, or have adverse side-effects.

Does PRP Work?

Although we tend to think of platelet-rich therapy as a relatively new development in medical treatment, platelet-rich plasma was developed back in the 1970s. It was first used in open heart surgery in 1987.[xv] Throughout the 1990s, the use of PRP to aid speedy recovery after surgery became more and more widespread.*xvi* In the mid-2000s, with almost two decades of surgical use and no reported adverse effects, some doctors were administering PRP therapy prior to surgery, in attempts to either strengthen the injured joint prior to surgery, or to pre-empt it altogether.

Studies on PRP have increased tremendously over the last decade. There are now double blinded studies showing safety & efficacy.

A 2006 study, "Treatment of chronic elbow tendinosis with buffered platelet-rich plasma,"*xvii* found that patients with chronic elbow tendonitis treated with a single PRP injection reported a 60% reduction in pain within eight weeks. Further improvements over time were recorded, with an 81% improvement after 6 months, and 91% improvement at the end of the study.

A further 5-year study, completed in 2014, confirmed the efficacy of PRP treatment on patients with chronic tennis elbow*xviii*. With an 83.9 success rate, the authors confirmed that, "clinically meaningful improvements were found in patients treated with leuko-cyte-enriched PRP."

Platelet-rich plasma, provides long-term pain relief, because it targets areas of injury and heals sources of injury. You might not get the potent anti-inflammatory effect that you would get with steroids right away. However, platelet-rich plasma has a more consistent trajectory of healing over time.

Lateral epicondylitis, also known as "tennis elbow," is one of the most common causes of upper extremity pain. It has various treatment options, including rest, oral medications, and commonly, steroid injections. Platelet-rich plasma offers a new, superior option for the treatment of tennis elbow.

In 2010, research led by Peerbooms et al was designed to determine the effectiveness of PRP compared with corticosteroid injections in patients with tennis elbow. It was concluded that "treatment of patients with chronic lateral epicondylitis with PRP reduces pain and significantly increases function, exceeding the effect of corticosteroid injection.

A more recent meta-analysis was published in the March 2017 issue of Arthroscopy by Dai et al. The analysis concluded that current evidence indicates that, compared with HA and saline, PRP injection in your knee joint may have more benefit in pain relief and functional improvement in patients with symptomatic knee osteoarthritis at 1 year post-injection.

With access to our certified laboratory and full-time scientists to process your blood, we are also able to tailor PRP, specifically for you and certain injury types. For instance, recent research has indicated that some injuries, such as muscle tears, would be better off being treated with Platelet-poor plasma[xix] and other injuries may require the PRP preparation to be "leukocyte-free." At Texas Cell Institute, we assess the final PRP preparation prior to injection to maintain the highest level of precision.

WHAT CONDITIONS DOES PRP TREAT?

Platelet-rich plasma can be used to treat a

wide range of musculoskeletal conditions and joint pain. It can be beneficial for many orthopedic injuries and in nearly all joints. The following is a list of common complaints that can benefit from platelet-rich plasma injection:

- ☑ Ligament Injuries
- ☑ Tendon Injuries
- ☑ Fasciitis
- ☑ Osteoarthritis
- ☑ Nerve Entrapment
- ☑ Chronic Low back pain
- ☑ Sciatica
- ☑ Temporomandibular joint (TMJ) syndrome - pain in the jaw joint

Patients may experience a spectrum of disorders on this list. Your physician will confirm the diagnosis and provide a list of all treatment options.

If you suffer from any of the above, or have a musculoskeletal injury that has not healed on its own and are suffering from pain that is limiting your activity, and want to know if PRP may be right for you, visit http://www.texascellinstitute.com. Use our 'Ask the Doctor' form to contact my team and I. We will be happy to evaluate you for PRP treatment and suggest a course of action that makes sense for your personal circumstances and condition.

How Can PRP Help Me?

If you have any kind of musculoskeletal condition with joint pain, the chances are your current treatment plan has been designed to mask the pain. As we have already seen, if you've been prescribed NSAIDs or narcotics, or had steroid injections, all those things have been used to try and make you comfortable, but not to deal with the underlying issues. You're on a path that could lead to costly medications, side effects, steroid-induced soft tissue degeneration, surgery, and ultimately chronic pain.

What PRP offers is an alternative that bridges the gap between true conservative options and surgery, in a way that's not focused on simply masking the pain, but on kick-starting regeneration.

Yes, PRP does offer pain relief, and it does help reduce inflammation. It does that not by cutting off the body's signal that it needs to heal, the way traditional painkillers do, but by delivering the materials needed for healing, quicker and in higher concentrations. It helps to heal sources of injury, and it allows a regeneration to occur, in areas where your normal bodies' capability failed you. With PRP, you are re-stimulating the bodies' own capability of healing injury.

So, the reasons that you should consider platelet-rich plasma over the traditional forms of therapy are that

a) it may be a superior form of therapy, giving better pain relief over the long term,

b) it doesn't include the harmful side-effects of over-the-counter, prescription, or narcotic drugs and steroid injections,

c) and it can help you avoid or delay surgery.

HOW DO I PREPARE FOR A PRP INJECTION?

PRP is defined as a simple same-day procedure, because everything is done during a single visit. It includes registration, check in, blood draw, blood processing, preparation, anesthesia, precise image-guided injection, nurse-directed recovery and discharge.

To give you an idea of what to expect, let's walk through the entire process from initial consultation to aftercare.

When you come to the initial consultation, we ask that you bring your imaging studies and reports that reflect your joint of injury.

It's also helpful if you can provide any recent bloodwork results & previous consultation and procedure notes from your current healthcare provider. On your first visit, we will talk to you, get to know your overall health, your specific injury, answer all your questions and educate you about your treatment options. We will discuss treatment options you have tried so far, and whether it has been effective or failed you.

If you are a good candidate, we will talk to you about PRP and how it can help your specific injury. We will explain what PRP is, and how it works, and outline the procedure itself, the post-injection phase, and the rehabilitative phase. It is not unusual for us to do a power point presentation with groups of our patients to give them an in depth understanding of this treatment option.

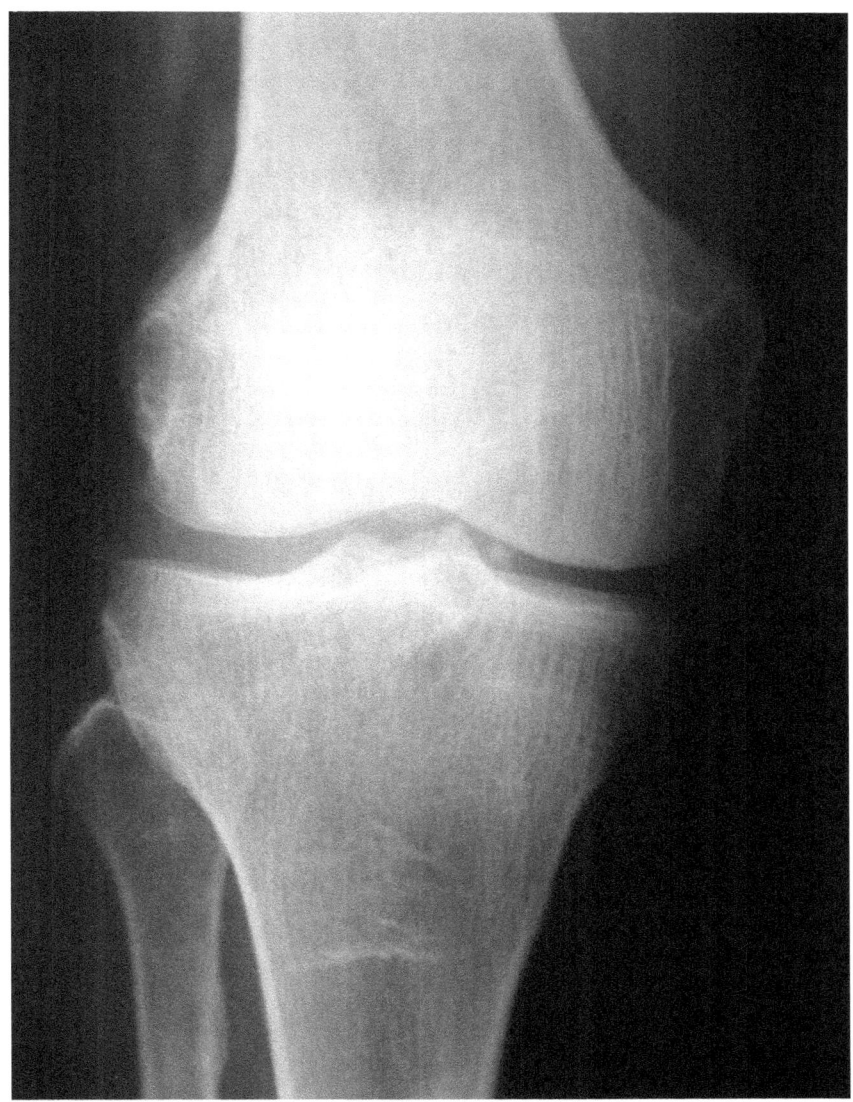

Figure 4: We will ask you to bring your medical imaging and results of any blood work on your first visit.

We take baseline bloodwork, to make sure there are no blood disorders that would be contra-indicators, such as low platelet count. We look at your current medication to identify anything like NSAIDs and blood thinners that would need to be stopped prior to treatment, after consultation with the prescribing doctor. We also review your imaging, and may do a diagnostic ultrasound.

Before you leave, we will put you on the Texas Cell Institute anti-inflammatory program, and give you a timeline for ceasing medication. We want to be your teammates in the journey toward healing. The only way we can do that is to empower you with the knowledge you need to understand the process.

Once you are satisfied that PRP is an option for you, you can schedule the procedure with our warm administrative staff. How long you must wait between the initial consultation and the procedure will depend on whether you need to stop blood-thinning medication, steroids or NSAIDs first and our current patient waiting list. On the day of procedure, you must avoid eating or drinking anything for eight hours prior to the procedure, as we give special importance to your comfort, safety and experience by providing you anesthesia.

WHAT IS THE PROCEDURE LIKE?

On the day of the procedure, you will check in and fill out the required paperwork. Once you are registered, you will change into a comfortable gown and be situated in our treatment suite. We will start an IV, and draw the blood for the platelet-rich plasma.

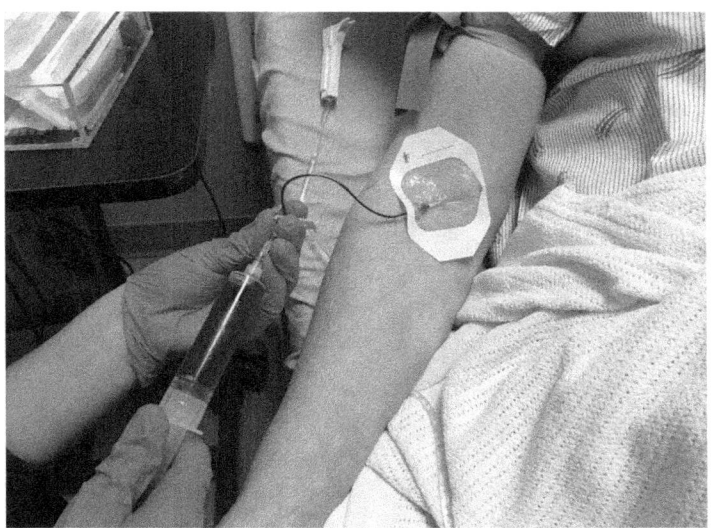

Figure 5: Drawing blood to create platelet-rich plasma

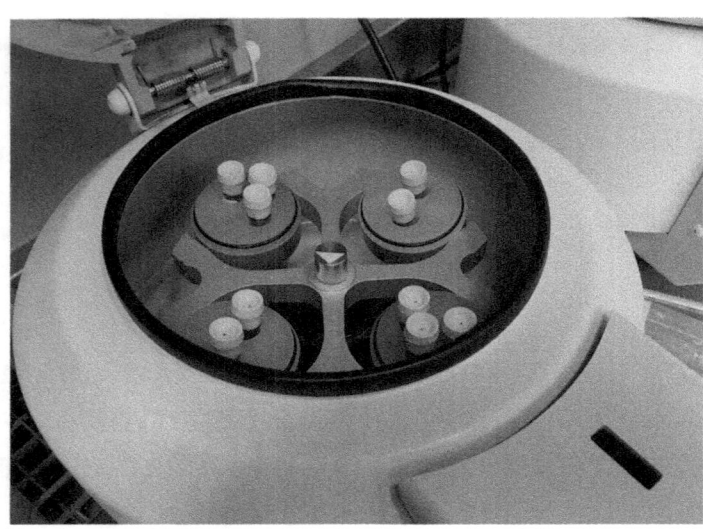

Figure 6: Your blood is centrifuged to sepa-rate the plasma and platelets from red and white blood cells.

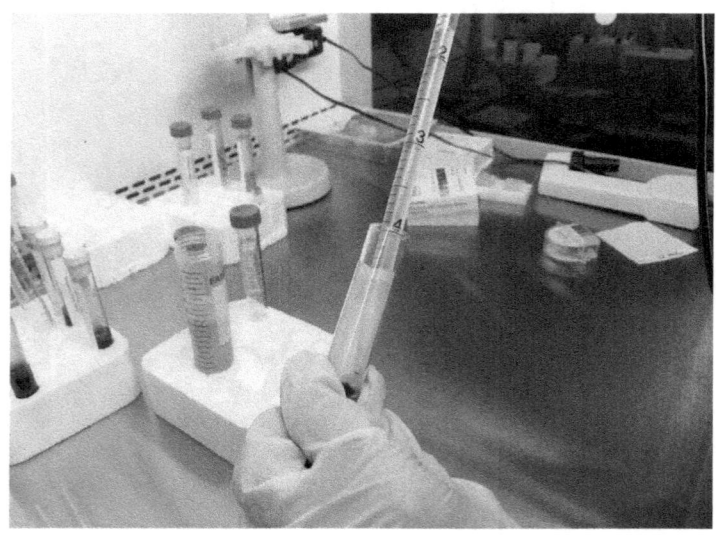

Figure 7: Drawing the platelet-rich plasma from the centrifuged solution.

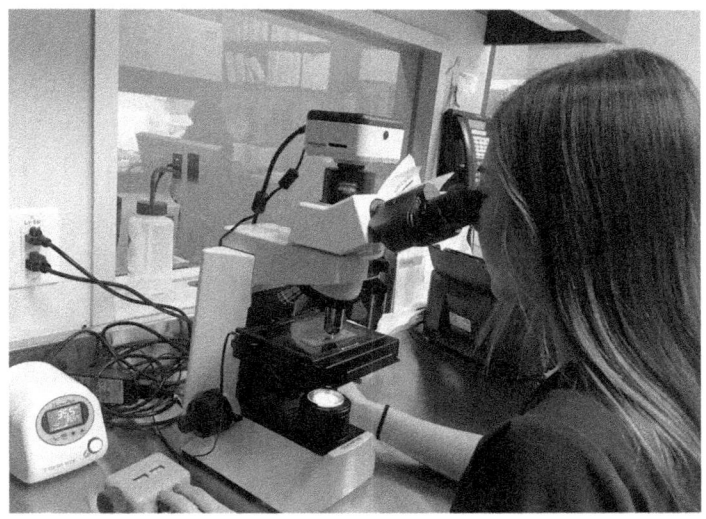

Figure 8: Checking the PRP under a microscope.

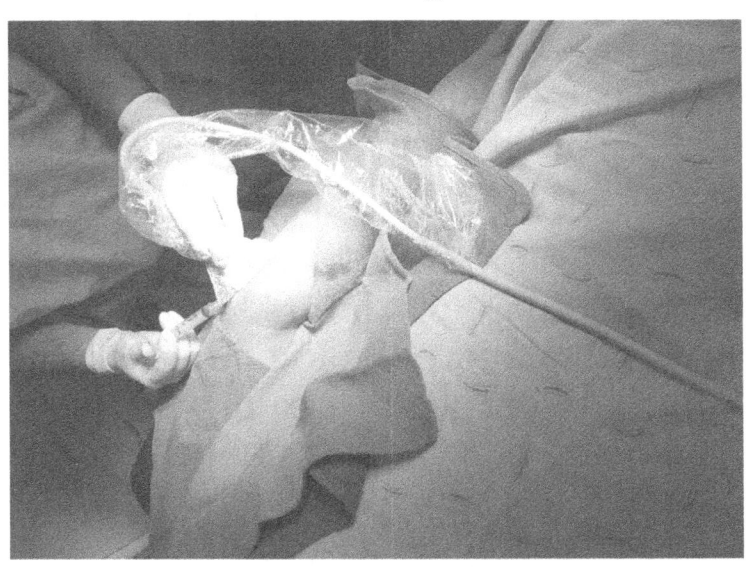

Figure 4: Injecting the PRP under image guidance.

Your blood is then taken to our FDA approved lab and processed. It is precisely centrifuged to separate and concentrate the platelets, and a microscopic analysis is completed to ensure everything is as it should be.

While your blood is being processed, we will talk to you, and answer any questions you have from your own research. I will explain again exactly what we are going to do, and talk you through the post-operative course.

Once the platelet-rich plasma has been precisely formulated, you are brought to the operating room by a nurse, comfortably in a stretcher. The nurse will hook you up to monitors, start oxygen going through your nose, and give you light intravenous sedation for your comfort.

When you are properly sedated, we will locate the area of injury, either using ultrasound or fluoroscopic guidance, or both. We prep and drape the area in a sterile fashion, numb the skin, and carefully perform the injection under image guidance.

Once injected, the activated platelets in the platelet-rich plasma unload growth factors and alert your body to send regenerative cells to the area of injury to help heal and regenerate damaged, non-healing tissue.

After the procedure, we then take you to the recovery room. You will be situated there, monitored by a nurse, and kept comfortable until you are safe to go home.

We have found that with anesthesia our patients tolerate PRP therapy very well. Patients may feel sore for one or two days after the procedure, which reflects the initiation of the inflammatory response. Often, patients don't feel any soreness. Our patients usually only need to take very mild analgesics during this time, if anything at all.

WHAT HAPPENS AFTER I RECEIVE PRP THERAPY?

The post-injection phase is co-managed with high-level physical therapists and functional rehabilitation specialists. It is our experience that proper rehabilitation after the procedure is critically important to optimize a successful outcome for you. You will be an important, active participant in your own rehabilitation and keep a journal of your daily exercises and resolution of symptoms.

We usually start with 3-7 days of rest. During this time, you will work on increasing your passive range of motion and stretching. You won't do any motions that are painful or hard on the joints, such as running, jumping or high-resistance exercises. You will only be able to resume daily activities that do not require high torque, turning, cutting, or pounding of the joint. You will be given specific, personalized instructions regarding rehabilitation after the PRP therapy.

After a week to 10 days, we initiate focused, high-quality physical therapy and functional rehabilitation with one of our recommended specialists. Under special circumstances for our patients that travel from long distances, we work closely with your existing or chosen therapist to ensure your progress is going as expected.

Healing will occur over the next 1-12 weeks and can continue even longer than that. It may take up to 4-6 weeks for your body to decrease inflammation and heal the injury to the point where you start to feel pain relief. Follow up will occur at 4-6 weeks after your procedure, at which point you will progress to the next stage of rehabilitation.

From this point, you will email me on a weekly basis with your progress, and any questions you might have. This ensures we remain active participants in your therapy, and helps us stay focused and on course with a decreased chance of any setbacks.

Depending on the level of damage or the site of the injury, you may only need one PRP injection. Although many patients have done well after one injection, those with moderate to severe issues may benefit synergistically from multiple injections to the area.

It is very important to understand that this treatment is not like cortisone, which provides a short, quick-fix. Platelet-rich plasma is part of a commitment to promote long-term healing. The process of PRP requires time and is coupled with individualized physical therapy and functional rehabilitation. You will see that PRP accelerates and strengthens the recovery process over time and gives you a better opportunity to get back to sport and activity without weakness, pain, and need for modification.

CONTRA INDICATORS AND COMPLICATIONS?

While Platelet-rich plasma therapy is perfectly safe for the clear majority of people, there are a few situations in which it is contraindicated. PRP would not be suitable for anyone with an abnormal initial platelet count, whether that's a high count (thrombocytosis) or a low one (thrombocytopenia). Similarly, anyone with a blood-clotting disorder, or any blood-borne disorder or active blood-borne cancer would pose high risks, and would be unsuitable for this kind of treatment.

There are also cases in which we would delay treatment until a potential threat is dealt with or subsides: such as ensuring patients are safely withdrawn from anti-platelet, anti-coagulant, or blood thinning medications; or waiting for a fever or infection to clear up.

Although it's extremely uncommon, the risks of platelet-rich plasma treatment include those associated with any injection including:

☑ Pain
☑ Infection
☑ Bleeding
☑ Nerve injury
☑ Skin discoloration

These risks are associated with the injection itself, rather than the PRP therapy. Remember, there is no risk of allergy, because you're getting your body's own cells back. The only risks related to PRP therapy are:

☑ no relief of symptoms
☑ worsening of symptoms

This might happen if you have been taking NSAIDs or narcotics to mask the pain and stop taking them prior to PRP therapy. There are also some people who, for as yet unknown reasons, simply don't respond to PRP therapy.

QUESTIONS TO ASK YOUR PRP THERAPY PROVIDER

If you are considering PRP Therapy, there are a few questions you should ask about both the physician carrying out the procedure, and the facility where it is undertaken.

ABOUT THE FACILITY

- ☑ Does your facility have a proper laboratory?
- ☑ Do the laboratory staff have expertise in cell preparation and analysis?
- ☑ Is the lab able to tailor the plasma concentrate to the injury to be treated per the physician's directions?
- ☑ How are these platelets prepared from beginning to end?
- ☑ How are the platelets qualified? How are

you making sure you're injecting me with properly prepared platelets? Or ensuring the PRP is not contaminated with red and white blood cells?

☑ Are you injecting PRP blindly or under image guidance?

☑ Are you injecting PRP in a sterile environment?

☑ What is the patient experience like?

☑ Are procedures carried out in a proper procedure suite or simply in a patient exam room?

ABOUT THE PHYSICIAN

☑ Will I receive end-to-end care from the same physician?

☑ Who will administer the injection? Will it be the physician, or a nurse or an assistant?

☑ Is the physician board certified?

☑ Does the physician have expertise in musculoskeletal pain management?

☑ Does the physician have clinical experience working under ultrasound and fluoroscopic guidance?

☑ What type of experience does your physician have with these injections?

THE TEXAS CELL INSTITUTE

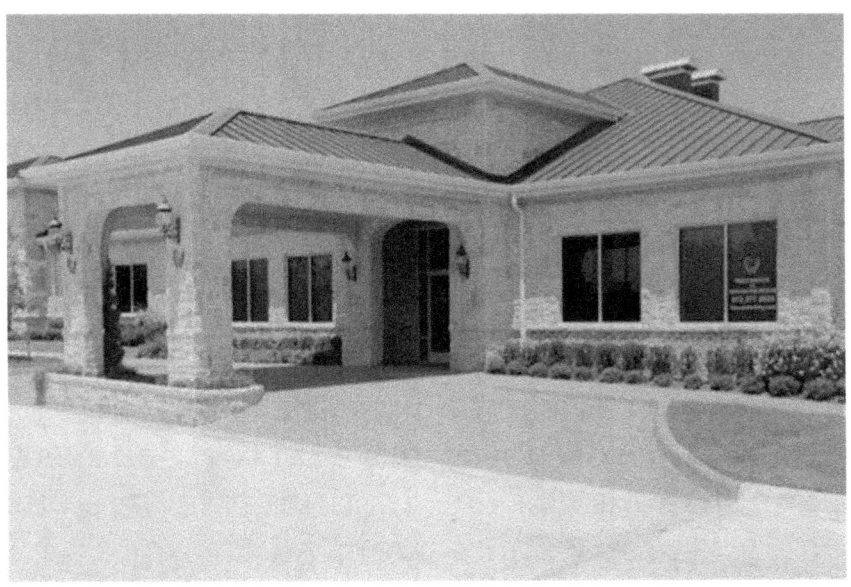

Figure 50: The Texas cell Institute, a pur-pose-built state-of-the-art facility.

The Texas Cell Institute for Regenerative Medicine was founded by myself, Dr. Amit Mirchandani, a double board-certified anes-thesiologist and pain management specialist

with a unique training in regenerative medicine, musculoskeletal and spine injury,
ultrasound and fluoroscopic guidance, and a
non-narcotic based philosophy.

I closely collaborate with Dr. Marius Meint-
jes, a PhD scientist whose background is in
cellular processing and technology. The collaboration has taken regenerative medicine
to the highest level.

Together, we offer the most advanced, non-
narcotic, non-surgical approaches to musculoskeletal injuries, utilizing cell therapy
techniques which enhance the body's own
natural abilities to heal in a state-of-the-art
facility complete with its own FDA certified
lab.

We are also able to analyze the cell count under the microscope and we do that for every
patient. At Texas Cell Institute, we give our
patients preparation details and a proper cell
count prior to the injection. Many clinics pre-
pare PRP therapy that doesn't work for
patients. Often, this is because the preparation methods are flawed and they skip the
analysis of the PRP before injecting their patients.

Our goal is to treat every one of our patients as a VIP, with the utmost attention to detail. Our staff at Texas Cell Institute take the time to get to know our patients and understand their injuries, questions and concerns, rather than rushing into treatment. They also take the time to understand the patient's goals, and consider the therapies already undergone, and their results.

We are not a "volume based" clinic, where you will see a waiting room filled with frustrated patients waiting for their 5-10 minutes with a physician or sometimes an assistant, only to leave confused and even more frustrated with a slew of prescriptions. We have established a practice where we are teammates in empowering you with treatment options most places can't begin to offer. We have created an unmatched experience for our patients where we limit the patients we see each day to make sure you remain the focus and epicenter our care.

COSTS INVOLVED AND INSURANCE

Currently, insurance providers consider platelet-rich plasma injection experimental.

What that means is, although the cost of the initial consultation, and the physical therapy and after-care components are generally covered, the cost of the procedure itself is not covered under insurance.

At Texas Cell Institute, we have an excellent financial advisory team that helps you navigate different payment options. In some circumstances, it may be possible to meet this cash component by accessing savings in a Health Savings Account (HAS), which are tax free savings account patients can use for their own health care costs. Our team will also work with patients to help them cover the cost, which may involve setting up a personalized payment plan. We also undertake work pro-bono, and we have even had one patient who paid for another patient's treatment, where we could pass on savings for both. Our goal is to ultimately help you and help you find a way to access this beneficial therapy.

At Texas Cell Institute, we have kept baseline costs for platelet-rich plasma therapy for our patients under $1,000 and that includes the facility cost, lab costs, and physician costs. Clinics with much lesser quality therapy and approaches often charge significantly more for PRP. Again, our goal is to help as many patients as possible have access to this therapy and ultimately help them avoid long-term medication, surgery, and a life of chronic, nagging pain.

At Texas Cell Institute, our mission is to reach everyone with chronic joint pain and offer the highest quality of regenerative medicine approaches. Until insurance companies come to their senses to fully cover PRP therapy, we will continue to offer it to patients at an affordable cost, and let them know it's not just a rich person's therapy. We want to be a solution for patients to ultimately heal their injuries, who need to save their money, who need to prevent surgery if possible, to save themselves from spending hard-earned money at the pharmacy every month; those are the people we seek to help.

That's why we have worked hard to keep the cost down, while offering treatment at the highest standards and not compromising on safety or quality.

WHAT OUR PATIENTS SAY

"Thank you for healing my arm! I am so grateful for your generosity and motivation for helping people. I feel so lucky to have the opportunity to have this procedure. It has changed my life! I can use my arm without pain and sleep at night.

Keep doing what you're doing."

-TG RN

"My Achilles was partially torn and I tried everything- multiple medications, narcotics, steroid injections, bracing. Nothing worked for me. I am a severe diabetic and my surgeon did not want to operate on me. I am grateful for my PRP procedure that took away the pain."

-MC

"I highly recommend Dr. Mirchandani and the Texas Cell Institute! I've never seen a staff so dedicated to ensuring patients receive the absolute best outcome possible! Hands down the best facility for PRP/stem cell therapy I have visited

-Dr. SM

I went to Dr. Mirchandani after ITB inflammation that has interfered with my running since 2013. I had a steroid injection back then with no benefit. I switched shoes and would K tape my knees to get through runs but I was no longer enjoying running due to the pain. I found Dr M to be an expert on PRP and that he had a wealth of information on stem cell therapy. We discussed all the options at length and I learned about the harmful effects of steroid injections. I had my PRP procedure done in early May 2016 and that constant nagging pain on the outside of the knee is no longer a barrier to my running!! Thank you Dr M and his wonderful staff for the quick and efficient care I received. I highly recommend PRP over steroid injections, for long lasting results using your own body's healing processes. And Dr. M and his facility has the ability to deliver viable platelet rich plasma under controlled conditions, into your tissues and ensure that there is a concentrated amount of activated platelets injected. And it feels very much like a steroid injection...minus the side-effects!

-ND

When I was in 8th grade, I busted my knee running the 200 during track practice. My spike got stuck in the block and when I took off, I fell and hit my knee on a concrete slab. After about a month of it getting worse, I had surgery. In the surgery, they found cartilage damage not shown on the MRI and I was told I couldn't run again. I had some relief, but a few months later the pain came back with popping. We went back to the doctor and they wanted to do another surgery. But one of our friends recommended we go to Dallas and check out Texas Cell Institute. So, we looked into it and set up an appointment. The doctors were extremely kind and wanted the best for me. After the first set of injections, I had a lot of relief but it was still a little painful. So, we set up another round of injections and I now have complete relief. Before the injections, I was told I couldn't ever run again. I ran for the first time in two and a half years with no pain. So, a special thanks goes out to Dr. Mirchandani and the whole team at Texas Cell Institute.

-JC

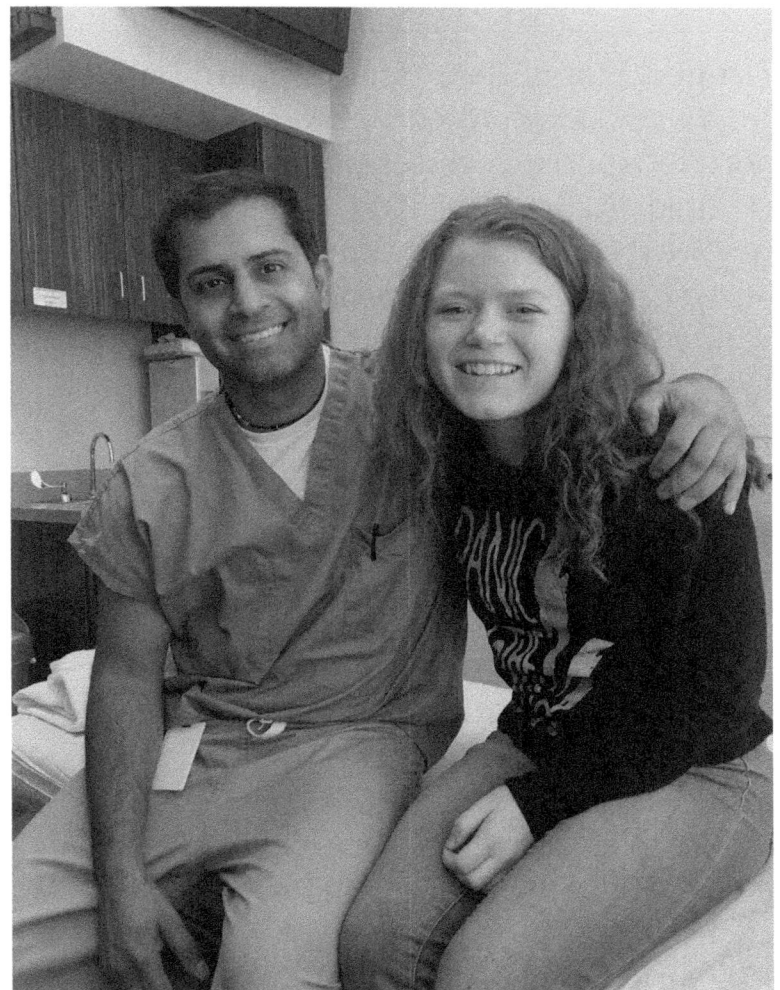

Figure 61: Dr Mirchandani with a patient after successful PRP therapy.

---

[i] (Andersson 2008)
[ii] (Centers for Medicare & Medicare Services 2014)

iii (United States Bone and Joint Initiative 2014, http://www.boneandjointburden.org/2014-report/ib0/prevalence-select-medical-conditions)
iv (United States Bone and Joint Initiative 2014, http://www.boneandjointburden.org/2014-report/xe1/cost-treat-musculoskeletal-diseases)
v (United States Bone and Joint Initiative 2014, http://www.boneandjointburden.org/2014-report/xe2/share-gdp)

vi (Mirkin and Hoffman 1978)
vii (Mirkin 2010)
viii (RO 1991)
ix (Drugabuse.Gov 2014)
x (Paulozzi, Budnitz and Xi 2006)
xi (Drugabuse.Gov 2015)
xii (- Pubmed - NCBI 2015)
xiii (Cardone and Tallia 2002)
xiv (Wernecke, Braun and Dragoo 2015)
(Ferrari, Zia and Valbonesi 1987;10)
xvi (Schwartz 2009)
xvii (Mishra and Pavelko 2006)
xviii (Mishra, et al. 2014)
xix (Dragoo 2016)

ABOUT THE AUTHOR

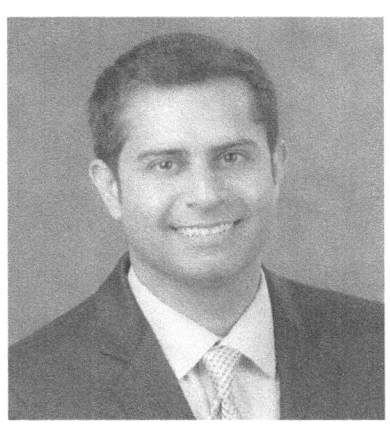 Dr Amit Mirchandani grew up in New Orleans and, from there, went to Memphis, TN, where he attended Rhodes College and the University of Tennessee College of Medicine as a Bland W. Cannon Scholar.

He completed his residency in anesthesia at Yale University and his fellowship in Interventional Pain Management at Rush University in Chicago.

During his fellowship, Dr. Mirchandani became passionate about pain management, and exploring alternative options for patients, which led to his move to Dallas, where he founded the Texas Cell Institute. He is double board-certified in both anesthesia and pain management.

Dr. Mirchandani had a simple desire when he founded Texas Cell Institute - to help his patients with joint pain get back to the life they want to live. Texas Cell Institute is designed as more than a typical pain practice that simply helps patients mask their painful symptoms for short periods of time. It is a regenerative medicine practice that focuses on utilizing autologous cells to help heal injury and give patients back their functionality. The goal is to not only reverse painful symptoms, but to help injuries heal.

Dr. Mirchandani is a pioneer in formulating new methodologies to harvest patient's own powerful regenerative cells and utilizing precise image guidance for delivery of these cells.

Dr. Mirchandani is a family man, a proud husband and father of two boys. He enjoys meeting new patients, traveling, reading, leadership development, playing basketball and New Orleans Saints football.

If you have a chronic nagging injury, neck pain, back pain, joint pain and have either hit a wall with the treatments you have tried or are trying to avoid them, call Texas Cell Institute today at 972-668-9612, or you can visit our website and contact us at www.texascellinstitute.com.

We look forward to helping you get back to the life you want to live.

BIBLIOGRAPHY

- Pubmed - NCBI. 2015. "An Evaluation Of Medications Commonly Used For Epidural Neurolysis Procedures In A Human Fibroblast Cell Culture Model." *Pubmed - NCBI.* December. http://www.ncbi.nlm.nih.gov/pubmed/21270726.

Andersson, Gunnar. 2008. *The Burden of Musculoskeletal Diseases in the United States: Prevalence, Societal and Economic Cost.* Rosemont, IL: American Academy of Orthopaedic Surgeons.

Cardone, Dennis A, and Alfred F Tallia. 2002. "Joint and Soft Tissue Injection." *Am Fam Physician,* July 15: 283-9.

Centers for Medicare & Medicare Services. 2014. *National health expenditure data.* May 5. Accessed December 1, 2015. https://www.cms.gov/Research-Statistics-Data-and-Systems/Statistics-Trends-and-Reports/NationalHealthExpendData/index.html.

Dragoo, Jason L. 2016. "The Use of Platelet-Rich and Platelet-Poor Plasma to Enhance Differentiation of Skeletal Myoblasts." *Orthopaedic Journal of Sports Medicine*, July.

Drugabuse.Gov. 2014. *America's Addiction To Opioids: Heroin And Prescription Drug Abuse.* May 14. https://www.drugabuse.gov/about-nida/legislative-activities/testimony-to-congress/2016/americas-addiction-to-opioids-heroin-prescription-drug-abuse.

—. 2015. *Overdose Death Rates.* December. https://www.drugabuse.gov/related-topics/trends-statistics/overdose-death-rates.

Ferrari, M, S Zia, and M Valbonesi. 1987;10. "A new technique for hemodilution, preparation of autologous platelet-rich plasma and intraoperative blood salvage in cardiac surgery." *International Journal of Artificial Organs* 47-50.

Mirkin, Gabe. 2010. *Dr. Gabe Mirkin on Health, Fitness and Nutrition. | Ice Delays Recovery from Injuries.* November 14. http://www.drmirkin.com/public/ezin e111410.html.

Mirkin, Gabe, and Marshall Hoffman. 1978. *The Sports Medicine Book.* Boston: Little Brown & Co.

Mishra, A K, N V Shrepnik, S G Edwards, G L Jones, S Samson, D A Vermillion, M L Ramsey, D C Karli, and A C Rettig. 2014. "Efficacy of platelet-rich plasma for chronic tennis elbow: a double-blind, prospective, multicenter, randomized controlled trial of 230 patients." *American Journal of Sports Medicine* 463-71.

Mishra, A, and T Pavelko. 2006. "Treatment of chronic elbow tendinosis with buffered platelet-rich plasma." *American Journal of Sports Medicine*

1174-8.

Paulozzi, L J, D S Budnitz, and Y Xi. 2006. "Increasing deaths from opioid analgesics in the United States." *Pharmacoepidemiol Drug Saf,* September: 618-27.

RO, Johnson. 1991. "The Problems And Pitfalls Of NSAID Therapy In The Elderly (Part I)." - *Pubmed - NCBI.* https://www.ncbi.nlm.nih.gov/pubmed/1794009.

Schwartz, A. 2009. "A Promisingn Treatment for Athletes in Blood." *New York Times.* February 17. Accessed August 23, 2016. http://www.nytimes.com/2009/02/17/17blood.htm.

United States Bone and Joint Initiative. 2014. *The Burden of Musculoskeletal Diseases in the United States (BMUS), Third Edition.* Rosemont, IL: United States Bone and Joint Initiative.

Wernecke, Chloe, Hilary J Braun, and Jason L Dragoo. 2015. "The Effect of Intra-articular Corticosteroids on Articular Cartilage." *Orthopaedic Journal of Sports Medicine*, May.

Yadav, R, S Y Kothari, and D Borah. 2015. "Comparison of Local Injection of Platelet Rich Plasma and Corticosteroids in the Treatment of Lateral Epicondylitis of Humerus." *Journal of CLinical and Diagnostic Research.*

www.ingramcontent.com/pod-product-compliance
Lightning Source LLC
Chambersburg PA
CBHW070050210526
45170CB00012B/652